Yoga Harmony: Transform Your Body, Mind, and Soul - Discover Inner Peace, Flexibility, and Strength for Every Body, Every Day."

Carol H Graham

Table of contents..

Introduction:

- The Yoga Way to Brilliance:

Introduction:

The Yoga Way to Brilliance

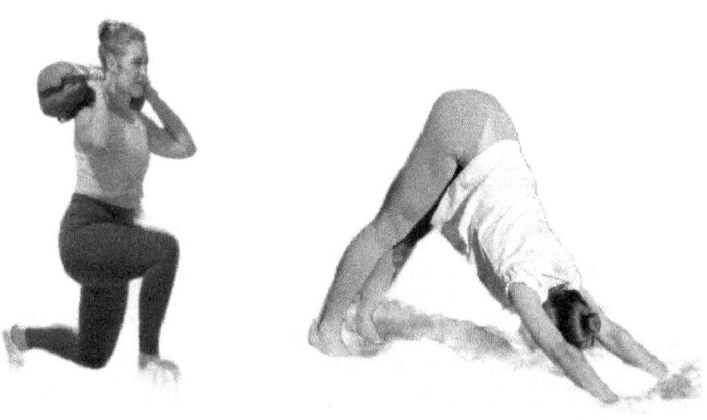

Leave on a journey of self-exposure and change with "The Yoga Way to Splendor."

- This book is your visa to opening your internal brightness and exploiting your endless potential.

In a world stacked up with humming about, yoga offers a place of refuge for both the body and mind.

"The Yoga Way to Magnificence" is your manual for this place of refuge, where you'll uncover the outdated understanding of yoga and its solid ability to illuminate your direction.

Yoga isn't just about broadening or winding your body into testing presents. A critical perspective feeds your soul and blends each piece of your reality in with splendor.

- The primary part takes you on a trip of self-exposure, igniting the glimmer inside you. It familiarizes you with the substance of yoga thinking and how it can transform you.

Breathing is life's most central show, and in the ensuing area, you'll become astounded at pranayama.

Examine the profundities of your breath, open vitality, and seat the presence force inside you.

This part outfits you with precious strategies to achieve mental clarity and genuine vitality through perceptive unwinding.

Asanas, or yoga presents, structure the bedrock of your preparation.

Segment three dives into these positions, preparing you to make serious solid areas for fortitude, flexibility, and harmony. From central positions to state of the art positions, you'll find how each asana adds to your outing towards brilliance.

- Versatility is crucial to each movement, and area four familiarizes you with yoga models for each body.

Regardless of your age or capacity level, you'll find addresses that suit your necessities and license you to embrace the full scope of your actual limit.

This book goes past the physical, hopping significantly into the exceptional mind-body relationship in area five.

You'll uncover how yoga updates mental thriving, directing strain, and creating interior amicability.

Supporting your body is likewise basic, and in segment six, you'll sort out some way to fuel your journey with yoga-blended sustenance.

- Find how your eating routine can upgrade your preparation and thriving:

"The Yoga Way to Splendor" isn't just about preparing on the mat; it's connected to embracing yoga in each piece of your life.

Section seven helps you on the most capable technique to make yoga an everyday custom, incorporating it into your day to day practice for persevering through benefits.

Yoga understands no age limits. Area eight reveals how yoga takes extraordinary consideration of kids, seniors, and in the center between, ensuring prosperity for all.

It acclimates to your specific necessities and offers an extensive method for managing aging gracefully.

Stress and torture are unavoidable in our lives, but segment nine outfits you with yoga's patching fixes.

Regulate pressure and decrease torture through yoga's thorough technique, resuscitating your inside wonder.

- As you progress in your yoga cycle, area ten examines the significant significance of yoga, taking you from the genuine asanas to light in standard everyday presence.

The outing doesn't end there. The finale of this book is connected to embracing the understanding inside, coinciding yoga's knowledge into your regular presence.

- Your yoga cycle is a dependable encounter of learning and improvement, and "The Yoga Way to Magnificence" is your well established companion.

With two comprehensive enhancements, this book outfits you with an instrument compartment for your yoga cycle, including recommended resources and a manual for yoga groupings redid to unequivocal targets.

- The record fills in as your aide, helping you with investigating the treasure trove of keenness held inside these pages.

Open your splendor and leave on a weighty journey with "The Yoga Way to Quality."
This book is your manual for embracing the full scope of your actual limit and pervading each piece of your reality with brightness. Your interaction starts here, where quality meets yoga.

Chapter 1:

Lighting Your
Internal Fire

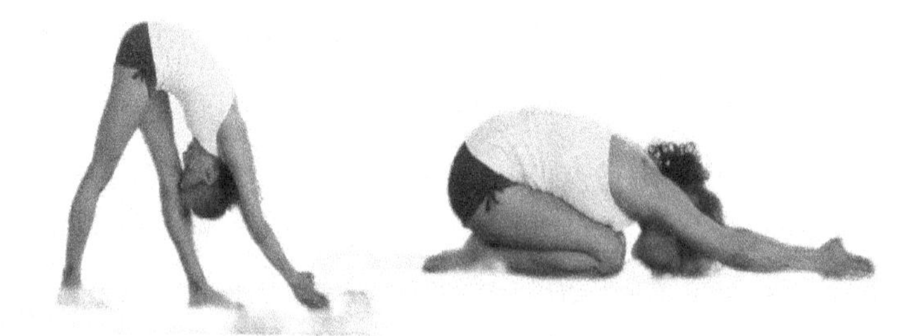

Getting Your Inner Fire going" is not simply a book; it's an excursion of tone- exposure and change.

Inside its runners lies the companion to opening your internal brilliance and taking advantage of the measureless depository of your true capacity.

- In a world that continually requests our consideration, this book offers you a hallowed space- a safe- haven for your body, psyche, and soul:

" Getting Your Inner Fire going" is your primer for this safe- haven, where you will reveal the antiquated sapience of yoga and its amazing capability to light your way to splendor.

Yoga is a commodity other than a factual exertion; a significant way of allowing feeds the factual quintessence of your being.

The book opens with a trip of tone- exposure, touching off the flash inside you.

It presents the center norms of yoga logic and uncovers how they can change your life into splendor.

Breathing, the substance of life itself, becomes the dominant focal point in the posterior part. Then, you'll excel at pranayama, the study of breath.

- Dig profound into your breath, open essentialness, and rig the actuality force inside you:

This section furnishes you with invaluable procedures to achieve internal simplicity and factual energy through conscious comforting.

Asanas, the factual stations of yoga, structure the underpinning of your training.

Part three is your passage to understanding these stations and how they help with creating areas of strength for solidarity, rigidity, and equilibrium.

From the central stations to the farther advanced bones you'll find the meaning of every asana on your way to brilliance.

- Rigidity is crucial on any excursion, and section four acquaints you with yoga models for each body:

Anyhow of your age or capability position, this part guarantees you find a product that lines up with your remarkable musts, permitting you to probe your outside capacity.

In any case, yoga is not just about factual capability; it dives into the extraordinary psyche body association, as delved in section five.

Then, you will uncover how yoga upgrades internal substance, empowering you to oversee pressure and develop internal harmony.

Also imperative is feeding your body, which is tended to in section six. You'll figure out how to fuel your excursion with yoga- implanted food.

This part clarifies how your eating routine can consolidate your training and by and large substance.

" Getting Your Inward Fire going" is about a commodity beyond training on the mat; it's tied in with embracing yoga in each point of your life.

- Section seven will direct you on the most complete system to make yoga an everyday custom, faultlessly integrating it into your diurnal practice for enduring advantages:

Yoga rises above age arrestment points, and part eight shows how it takes special care of everybody, from children to seniors, guaranteeing health for all.

It adjusts to your particular conditions and offers an all encompassing way to deal with perfecting with age.

- Life surely presents pressure and agony, yet section nine outfits you with yoga's mending cures:

You will figure out how to oversee pressure and ease torment through yoga's comprehensive methodology, reviving your internal brilliance.

As you progress in your yoga process, part ten dives into the unearthly depth of yoga, taking you from the factual asanas to edification in regular diurnal actuality.

- Be that as it may, the excursion does not end there:

The book's homestretch is tied in with embracing the concordance outside, faultlessly entrapping yoga's sapience into your everyday presence.

Your yoga process is a deep confirmed experience of literacy and development, and" Getting Your Inner Fire going" is your long lasting friend.

- With two complete supplements, this book gives you a tool store for your yoga process, including specified means and a primer for yoga relations custom fitted to unequivocal objects:

The record fills in as your companion, aiding you with exploring the mama burden of sharpness held inside these runners.

Open your splendor and set out on a groundbreaking excursion with" Getting Your Inner Fire going.

" This book is your primer for embracing the full range of your true capacity and implanting each part of your actuality with brilliance.

Your process begins then, where your inner fire meets the splendor of yoga.

2. Discharge Your Inside Yogi:

A Trip of Self-Disclosure" is in excess of a book; it's an odyssey into the profundities of your being, a groundbreaking excursion that opens your inward brilliance and reveals the limitless potential that dwells inside you.

In reality as we know it, where interruptions proliferate and the speed of life appears to be unrelenting, this book offers you a hallowed shelter — a safe-haven for your body, psyche, and soul.

- "Discharge Your Inside Yogi" fills in as your compass, directing you through this safe-haven and uncovering the old insight of yoga, which has the uncommon ability to light your way to brightness.

Yoga isn't just an actual practice; a significant way of thinking feeds the center of your reality.

The book starts with an investigation of self, touching off the flash of mindfulness inside you. It acquaints you with the center standards of yoga reasoning, enlightening how they can change your life into brightness.

- Part two becomes the dominant focal point as you dig into the craft of pranayama, the study of breath — the actual embodiment of life. I

in this part, you'll become amazing at cognizant breathing, opening imperativeness and bridling the existence force inside you.

These significant strategies award you mental clearness and actual dynamic quality.

Asanas, the actual stances of yoga, are uncovered in part three. You will comprehend how they structure the foundation of your work on, giving areas of strength for solidarity, adaptability, and equilibrium.

From basic stances to further developed ones, you'll find the meaning of every asana on your way to splendor.

Adaptability is principal on any excursion, and part four acquaints you with yoga presents reasonable for each body.

- Regardless of your age or expertise level, this section guarantees you find representatives that resound with your exceptional requirements, permitting you to investigate your maximum capacity.

In any case, yoga isn't exclusively about actual ability. It dives into the groundbreaking brain body association, as investigated in part five.

- This part uncovers how yoga upgrades mental prosperity, preparing you to oversee pressure and develop inward harmony.

Similarly fundamental is sustaining your body, a subject investigated in section six.
You'll figure out how to fuel your excursion with yoga-imbued sustenance, understanding how your eating routine can intensify your training and generally speaking prosperity.

"Discharge Your Inner Yogi" is about something beyond a training on the mat; it's tied in with meshing yoga into each feature of your life.

- Part seven offers direction on the most proficient method to make yoga a day to day custom, flawlessly integrating it into your everyday practice for enduring advantages.

Yoga realizes no age cutoff points, and section eight exhibits how it takes special care of everybody, from children to seniors, guaranteeing health for all.

It adjusts to your particular requirements and offers an all encompassing way to deal with improving with age.

Life definitely presents pressure and torment, yet part nine outfits you with yoga's mending cures.

You'll figure out how to oversee pressure and ease torment through yoga's all encompassing methodology, reviving your inward brightness.

- As you advance on your yoga process, part ten digs into the otherworldly profundity of yoga, taking you from the actual asanas to edification in regular daily existence.

In any case, the excursion doesn't finish up there. The book's finale is tied in with embracing the amiability inside, consistently meshing yoga's insight into your everyday presence.

- Your yoga process is a long lasting experience of learning and development, and "Delivery Your Inward Yogi" is your deep rooted buddy.

With two thorough indices, this book gives you a tool compartment for your yoga process, including prescribed assets and a manual for yoga successions custom-made to explicit objectives.

- The list fills in as your guide, assisting you with exploring the gold mine of shrewdness held inside these pages.

Open your brightness and set out on a groundbreaking excursion with "Delivery Your Inner Yogi."

- This book is your manual for embracing the full range of your true capacity and injecting each part of your existence with brilliance.

Your process begins here, where your interior yogi meets the splendor of self-disclosure.

3. Lighting the Glimmer The Quintessence of Yoga Reasoning:

In a world overflowing with disarray and consistent development, "Lighting the Blaze: The Quintessence of Yoga Reasoning" is a signal of shrewdness, offering an impression, yet a significant submersion into the actual center of yoga's old way of thinking.

Inside these pages, the creator, whose energy for yoga reasoning is substantial, unwinds the well established bits of insight that have directed innumerable searchers on their otherworldly excursions.

- An Excursion of Self-Revelation:

"Lighting the Glimmer" rises above a simple clarification of yoga reasoning; it's an entry to self-disclosure and inward change.

The book's central goal is to assist perusers with leaving on a journey inside themselves, investigating the most profound openings of their spirits.

Yoga Past the Mat

Yoga is frequently inseparable from actual stances, however its actual pitch reaches out a long ways past the mat.

The writer splendidly uncovers the multi-layered parts of yoga reasoning, taking pursers on an excursion that investigates its moral standards, shrewdness lessons, and the functional use of these standards in day to day existence.

- Lucidity In the midst of Intricacy:

The way of thinking of yoga can be mind boggling, however "Lighting the Glimmer" is a reference point of lucidity in this intricacy.

It makes an interpretation of significant ideas into available information, making the lessons of yoga logicians interesting and pertinent to the cutting edge world.

- An Agreeable Mix of Old and Contemporary:

The book flawlessly mixes old insight with contemporary pertinence. It overcomes any barrier between yoga's ageless way of thinking and its down to earth utility in our feverish, innovation driven lives.

- Arousing Cognizance:

Through an investigation of yoga reasoning, perusers are welcome to stir their awareness and reveal the inactive potential inside. It's an excursion of self-acknowledgement, a course of figuring out one's motivation and spot in the universe.

- Your Internal Light:

"Lighting the Glimmer" is an update that the illumination of understanding dwells inside.

It's an encouragement to light that inward fire of intelligence and information, directing pursuers towards an existence of satisfaction, reason, and congruence.

This book isn't simply a philosophical investigation, but a groundbreaking aide, enlightening the way to a daily routine that is experienced, yet genuinely experienced.

"Lighting the Glimmer" is your visa to a more profound comprehension of the philosophical underpinnings of yoga, a guide to self-disclosure, and a challenge to embrace a day to day existence loaded up with shrewdness, reason, and light.

Chapter 2:

Breath of Life

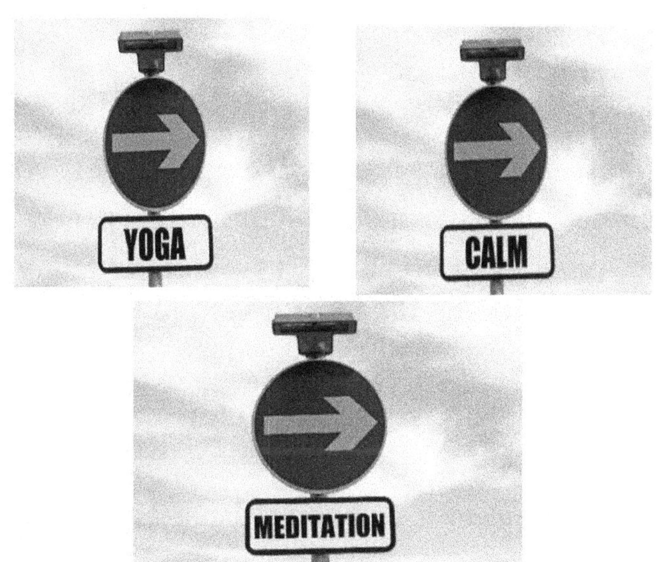

- Dominating Pranayama for Imperativeness:

In the steady hurrying around of current life, where stress spins out of control and energy is by all accounts in ceaselessly short stock, the old insight of Pranayama is a life saver.

- "Breath of Life:

Dominating Pranayama for Essentialness" is your far reaching manual for opening the existence force inside you, permitting you to saddle unfathomable imperativeness through the force of breath.

- The Breath: Your Door to Imperativeness.

Breath is in excess of a compulsory activity; it's the way to revive your whole existence.

"Breath of Life" strips back the layers of antiquated yogic insight, uncovering how cognizant breath control through Pranayama can stir your torpid energy and flood your existence with imperativeness.

- Fitting Life Energies:

Pranayama is the craft of adjusting the multifaceted snare of life energies, or prana, inside your body.

This book is your tutor on the excursion of reestablishing balance to these powers, prompting a newly discovered feeling of prosperity and unfathomable essentialness.

- Stress The board and Mental Clearness:

In a world loaded up with pressure and steady mental jabber, Pranayama is your safe-haven for serenity and mental lucidity.

This book acquaints you with strategies that calm the psyche, diminish pressure, and develop profound flexibility, all by basically saddling the force of your breath.

- Actual Restoration and Wellbeing:

Breath is life, and cognizant breathing is your key to actual restoration. "Breath of Life" investigates how Pranayama upgrades actual wellbeing, helps flow, and helps your body's regular detoxification processes.

It's a pathway to reestablishing and keeping up with prosperity from the back to front.

- Arousing the Profound Association:

Pranayama rises above the physical and mental; an otherworldly practice interfaces you to the significant profundities of your internal identity.

This book acquaints you with the profound element of breath, directing you on an extraordinary excursion of self-revelation and internal arousing.

- A Day to day existence in Equilibrium Is standing by:

"Breath of Life" isn't just a manual for Pranayama; it's an encouragement to carry on with an existence in wonderful equilibrium.

It's an update that the doorway to essentialness, lucidity, and profound arousing is the very breath you underestimate consistently.

This book is your identification to a day to day existence improved by energy, mental lucidity, and internal harmony.

Something beyond an aide, "Breath of Life" is your guide to dominating Pranayama, a deep rooted practice with the possibility to enlighten each feature of your reality.

It's a challenge to stir the power inside your breath and embrace a daily existence overwhelmed by essentialness, clarity, and tranquility.

Your excursion to dominating Pranayama and encountering endless imperativeness starts here.

2. Take In, Shimmer Out: The Force of Pranayama:

In the tireless twirl of life's requests, where stress and disarray frequently rule, the old insight of Pranayama arises as a guide of serenity and internal strength. "Take In, Shimmer Out:

The Force of Pranayama" is your exhaustive manual for tackling the significant force of breath to revive your body, brain, and soul.

- The Substance of Pranayama:

Pranayama isn't recently controlled breathing; it's the actual substance of life itself.

"Take In, Shimmer Out" discloses the enchantment of Pranayama, a training that holds the possibility to change your whole existence.

It's an encouragement to dig into the insight of the breath and find the wellspring of imperativeness inside you.

- Adjusting Life Energies:

Pranayama is the craft of orchestrating the existence energies, known as prana, inside your body.

This book fills in as your directing light on the excursion to reestablish balance to these powers, reviving a feeling of prosperity that emanates essentialness.

- Stress Authority and Mental Clearness:

In a world overflowing with interruptions and tensions, Pranayama is your desert spring of quietness and mental lucidity.

"Take In, Shimmer Out" presents procedures that quiet the brain, lessen pressure, and sustain profound versatility, all through the groundbreaking force of careful relaxing.

- Actual Rejuvenation and Wellbeing:

Breath isn't simply an actual demonstration; it's your life saver to a reestablished body.

This book enlightens how Pranayama upgrades actual prosperity, reinforces flow, and helps the body's regular detoxification processes.

It's your way to actual reestablishment and all encompassing wellbeing from the back to front.

- Otherworldly Association and Inward Arousing:

Past the physical and the psychological, Pranayama is a profound practice.

This book acquaints you with the significant otherworldly components of breath, directing you on an excursion of self-revelation, inward arousing, and association with the most profound openings of your spirit.

- Balance Looks for You:

"Take In, Shimmer Out" isn't simply an aide; it's a challenge to have an existence of significant equilibrium, imperativeness, and internal harmony.

It's an update that the way to prosperity, lucidity, and otherworldly arousing dwells inside your actual breath.

This book is your pass to a day to day existence suffused with unlimited energy, smartness, and peaceful tranquility.

In addition to an aide, "Take In, Shimmer Out" is your guide to dominating Pranayama, an immortal practice with the possibility to enlighten each part of your reality.

It's your challenge to stir the power inside your breath and embrace a daily existence loaded up with imperativeness, lucidity, and inward brilliance.

Your excursion to dominating Pranayama and encountering unlimited imperativeness starts here.

Chapter 3:

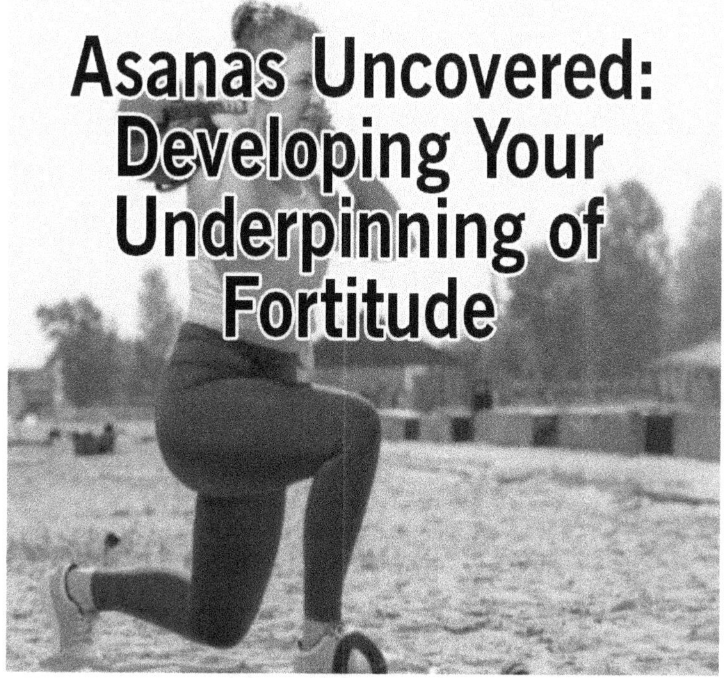

Amidst life's persevering turmoil and disturbance, we as a whole long for a strong groundwork to remain upon.

"Asanas Revealed: Developing Your Underpinning of Fortitude" is your widely inclusive manual for laying out an unshakable foundation through the act of yoga asanas, or stances.

- The Core of Asanas:

Asanas are not just actual activities; they are the actual heart of yoga, offering significant insight and essentialness to the people who embrace them.

"Asanas Unveiled" strips back the layers of these stances, uncovering their profound importance in developing actual strength as well as mental and close to home flexibility.

- An Excursion of Self-Disclosure:

Yoga asanas go past actual development; they are a way of self-disclosure.

This book is your directing light on an excursion inside, investigating the unpretentious subtleties of your body and the strength concealed inside.

It's an encouragement to comprehend and invigorate your establishment, both on and off the mat.

- Actual Strength and Equilibrium:

The asanas are your entryway to actual strength and equilibrium.

"Asanas Uncovered" dives into the specialty of adjusting strength, adaptability, and steadiness, giving a guide to a sound and strong body.

Through these stances, you'll track down actual power as well as an engaged brain and soul.

- Close to home Versatility and Prosperity:

Asanas are a way to sustain close to home strength and prosperity.

The book offers experiences close to home delivery that can go with the act of asanas, assisting you with overseeing pressure and accomplish profound balance.

- Careful Living Past the Mat:

"Asanas Revealed" doesn't stop at the mat; it stretches out to each feature of your life.

The standards learned in the act of asanas can be applied in your everyday encounters, directing you towards careful living, prosperity, and inward strength.

- An Existence of Equilibrium and Strength Is standing by:

"Developing Your Groundwork of Fortitude" isn't simply an aide; it's a challenge to have an existence of equilibrium, strength, and versatility.

It's an update that your establishment isn't simply the actual ground underneath you however the profound internal strength that upholds you notwithstanding life's difficulties.

Something beyond an aide, "Asanas Unveiled" is your guide to excelling at asanas.

It's your challenge to open the physical and profound strength that lives inside you, making ready for an existence of essentialness, balance, and relentless internal power.

Your excursion to developing your underpinning of fortitude starts here.

## 2.	Building	Blocks	of	Harmony:	The Underpinning of Yoga"

In a universe of consistent development and constant change, accomplishing a feeling of harmony appears to be a far off dream.

However, inside the pages of "Building Blocks of Harmony:
The Underpinning of Yoga," you'll find the antiquated insight that holds the way to adjust and quietness in your life.

- The Substance of Yoga's Establishment:

Yoga isn't just about bending your body into complex stances; it's tied in with laying out a strong groundwork of equilibrium in your life.

This book takes you on an excursion to uncover the key standards of yoga, the structure hinders that give the consistent ground to a reasonable, amicable presence.

- Physical and Mental Equilibrium:

"Building Blocks of Harmony" acquaints you with the fundamental yoga stances and rules that develop actual equilibrium.

In any case, it doesn't stop there; it proceeds to investigate how these stances convert into mental balance, assisting you with finding the serenity you've been looking for.

- Mind-Body Association:

The psyche and body are personally connected, and yoga is the extension that associates them.

This book discloses the force of the brain body association, showing the way that it very well may be bridled to make a day to day existence set apart by concordance, tranquility, and satisfaction.

- The Craft of Relaxing:

Breath is the groundwork of yoga, and in "Building Blocks of Harmony," you'll get familiar with the craft of cognizant relaxation.

Pranayama, or breath control, turns into a pathway to inward adjustment, a device for diminishing pressure, and a method for tracking down mental lucidity.

- Comprehensive Prosperity:

Yoga isn't simply an actual practice; it's a lifestyle. This book features how yoga standards stretch out past the mat, affecting your everyday decisions, your collaborations, and your relationship with the world.

It's an all encompassing way to deal with prosperity, cultivating actual wellbeing as well as mental, profound, and otherworldly prosperity.

- A Daily existence in Equilibrium Is standing by:

"Building Blocks of Harmony" isn't simply an aide; it's a challenge to carry on with an existence set apart by equilibrium and serenity.

It's an update that balance is certainly not an out of reach dream yet a substantial reality ready to be capable.

This book is your visa to a daily existence improved by equilibrium, congruity, and a significant association between your brain and body.

Something beyond a prologue to yoga's primary standards, "Building Blocks of Harmony" is a guide to making a day to day existence portrayed by equilibrium, serenity, and satisfaction.

It's a challenge to leave on an excursion of self-disclosure and all encompassing prosperity that will lead you to a daily existence in wonderful balance.

Your excursion to building a strong starting point for a healthy lifestyle starts here.

3. Building Blocks of Balance The Imaginativeness of Asanas"

In a world that continually challenges our feeling of equilibrium and soundness, the act of yoga asanas arises as a significant work of art. "

- Building Blocks of Balance The Masterfulness of Asanas" is your conclusive primer for dominating the indefectible stations of yoga, making an underpinning of physical, internal, and close to home harmony:

The Verse of Asanas Yoga asanas are further than factual conditioning; they're the verse of the body, an ensemble of solidarity and effortlessness.

" Building Blocks of Balance " discloses the imaginativeness natural in each posture, uncovering the significant sapience covered inside their swish excellence. An Excursion of tone- disquisition Yoga asanas aren't simple factual stations;

- They're a pathway to tone- disquisition. This book is your confident chum on a trip outside, permitting you to probe the complications of your body and the consonance it can negotiate:

It's a challenge to comprehend and brace your establishment, both on and off the yoga mat. Factual Dominance and Balance The asanas are your way to factual dominance and balance.

" Building Blocks of Harmony" dives into the perplexing equilibrium of solidarity, rigidity, and polish, offering direction for a body that is not a major area of strength for just nimbleness.

Through these stations, you will uncover factual essentialness as well as a protean psyche and soul.

Profound Inflexibility and Tranquility Asanas aren't just about factual capability; they support close to home inflexibility and internal tranquility.

- This book gives gests into the profound delivery and quiet that goes with the act of asanas, aiding you with overseeing pressure and achieving close to home balance:

Rising above the Mat " Asanas are not confined to the yoga mat; they stretch out to the total of your reality.

The norms learned in the act of asanas can be applied in your everyday actuality, encouraging factual essentialness as well as a feeling of harmony in all corridors of life.

A diurnal actuality in awful Equilibrium Is standing by " Building Blocks of Harmony" is not simply an assistant;

it's a challenge to have an actuality set piecemeal by balance, strength, and a bent feeling of balance.

It's an update that your establishment reaches out past the factual ground underneath you — it's the significant equilibrium that you convey outside, supporting you in exploring life's difficulties with effortlessness and strength. commodity beyond an assistant,"

- Building Blocks of Balance" is your companion to outstripping at asanas:

It's your challenge to find the tastefulness and power that live inside you, preparing for a diurnal reality loaded up with essentialness, balance, and an unshakeable inward harmony.

Your excursion to getting amazing at asanas and encountering awful balance starts then.

Chapter 4:

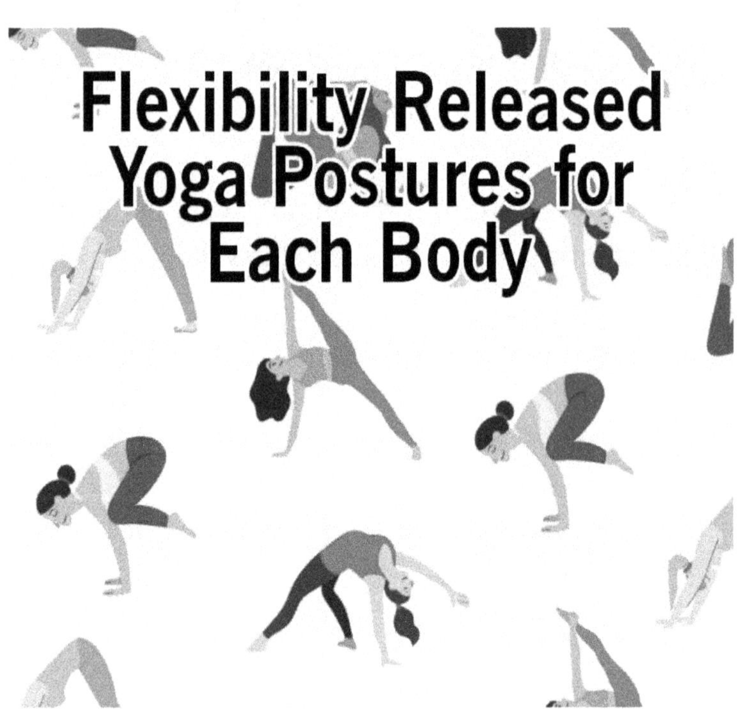

Flexibility Released Yoga Postures for Each Body

In a world that praises variety, inclusivity, and distinction, yoga is no exemption.

"Flexibility Released: Yoga Stances for Each Body" is your definitive manual for the act of yoga, accentuating that it is genuinely for each body, paying little mind to mature, shape, or wellness level.

- An Excursion of Inclusivity:

Yoga isn't a training restricted to the adaptable and the fit; it's a comprehensive excursion for each body.

"Versatility Released" praises the variety of human structures and the flexibility of yoga to meet every remarkable need.

- Custom fitted for All:

This book divulges yoga represents that are open and versatile for a large number of bodies.

Whether you are a novice or an accomplished yogi, whether you have actual constraints or are in top state of being, "Versatility Released" furnishes you with postures and varieties that can be custom-made to suit your particular prerequisites.

- A Range of Potential outcomes:

Yoga presents are not one-size-fits-all; they are a range of potential outcomes.

"Flexibility Released" urges you to investigate the rich woven artwork of yoga stances, finding the varieties that suit your body best.

It's an encouragement to break free from the imperatives of an unbending practice and embrace the smoothness of flexibility.

- Actual Wellbeing and Adaptability:

Yoga is an amazing asset for upgrading actual wellbeing and adaptability.

This book dives into representations that take care of all levels, from delicate stretches that elevate adaptability to additional difficult asanas that cultivate strength.

It's an excursion of actual essentialness and prosperity, open to all.

 • Profound Reverberation and Self-assurance:

Past the physical, "Flexibility Released" recognizes the profound reverberation of yoga.

It gives a protected and steady space for people, all things considered, to improve their fearlessness and close to home prosperity through the act of yoga.

 • A Training for Each Body:

"Asanas Released" rises above the possibility of yoga as an actual practice and positions it as a comprehensive way to deal with prosperity for each body.

This book is your manual for a training that adjusts to your exceptional body, your interesting requirements, and your extraordinary excursion.

It's an encouragement to find the boundless versatility of yoga, releasing its ability to upgrade your physical, close to home, and mental prosperity, paying little mind to what your identity is or where you're beginning from.

"Flexibility Released Yoga Postures for Each Body" is your own identification to a yoga practice that commends the lovely variety of the human experience.

Your excursion to flexibility, inclusivity, and prosperity starts here.

2. Versatility for All: Stances for Each Age and Capacity Level"

In this present reality where the quest for prosperity and imperativeness knows no age or actual restriction, "Flexibility for All:

Stances for Each Age and Capacity Level" remains as a signal of inclusivity and strengthening.

This far reaching guide rethinks yoga, making it available to people of each and every age and capacity.

- A Comprehensive Excursion:

Yoga is certainly not a select club for the youthful and adaptable; it's a widely inclusive excursion for everybody.

"Versatility for All" is a festival of the variety of human experience, stressing that yoga exceeds all logical limitations.

- Modified for Each Body:

This book disentangles the wealth of yoga stances, offering varieties and variations to take special care of various age gatherings and capacity levels.

Whether you're a kid, a senior, a fledgling, or somebody with actual restrictions, "Flexibility for All" gives a customized way to deal with your exceptional necessities.

- A Vast expanse of Stances:

Yoga stances are not static; they are a vast expanse of conceivable outcomes.

This guide welcomes you to investigate the huge range of yoga asanas, changing them to your remarkable body and capacity level. It's a call to break liberated from unbending assumptions and embrace the versatility inborn in yoga.

- Actual Wellbeing and Versatility:

Yoga is an intense device for improving actual wellbeing and versatility, and "Flexibility for All" is your vital aspect for opening its advantages.

From delicate stretches that elevate adaptability to altered representations that cultivate strength, this book upholds the prosperity of each and every age gathering and capacity level.

- Close to home Prosperity and Self-Acknowledgment:

Past the physical, yoga sustains close to home prosperity and self-acknowledgement.

"Versatility for All" recognizes the profound profundity of yoga, giving a safe and supporting space for people to upgrade fearlessness, close to home flexibility, and internal harmony, no matter what their age or actual limit.

- A Training for All Ages and Capacities:

"Flexibility for All" reclassifies yoga, making it a training for all ages and capacities.

It reaches out past actual stances, enveloping the all encompassing prosperity of psyche, body, and soul.

It is a demonstration of the flexibility of yoga and its ability to serve each person.

This book is your encouragement to investigate the unlimited flexibility of yoga, releasing its capability to improve your physical, profound, and mental prosperity, no matter what your age or state of being.

- "Versatility for All:

Stances for Each Age and Capacity Level" is your own manual for a yoga practice that embraces the variety of human experience.

Mind Over Issue The Force of Yoga

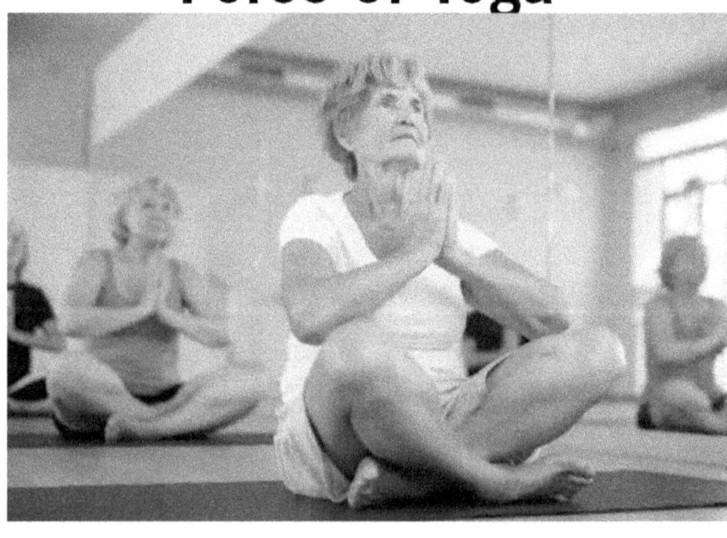

In the frantic speed of present day life, where the psyche frequently feels like a war zone, "Cerebrum Over Issue:

The Force of Yoga" arises as a directing light. This extensive aid divulges the noteworthy impact of yoga on the cerebrum, a training that engages you to recover dominance over your psychological and profound prosperity.

- The Brain Body Association:

Yoga isn't simply an actual practice; it's a significant excursion into the interconnectedness of the brain and body.

"Mind Over Issue" dives profound into this association, uncovering the unpredictable manners by which yoga can rework and restore your cerebrum.

- An Excursion of Care:

Yoga fills in as an amazing asset for developing care, the craft of being completely present at the time.

This book is your confidant friend on an excursion of self-disclosure, arousing your mindfulness, and permitting you to tackle the undiscovered possibility of your brain.

- Profound Strength and Stress Decrease:

In a world overflowing with stressors, yoga gives a safe-haven close to home versatility.

"Mind Over Issue" acquaints you with yoga's capacity to oversee pressure, develop profound prosperity, and cultivate close to home flexibility. It's a pathway to a quiet and focused profound state.

- Upgraded Mental Capability and Clearness:

Yoga doesn't simply quiet the psyche; it hoists mental capability and mental lucidity.

The book investigates how yoga can hone your intellectual capacities, support fixation, and enhance imaginative reasoning.

- Entryway to a mind's capabilities at its pinnacle:
- Mind Wellbeing and Brain adaptability:

Yoga isn't just about mental prosperity; it's about mind wellbeing.

"Mind Over Issue" uncovers the manners by which yoga upholds brain adaptability, the cerebrum's ability to adjust and revamp itself.

- It's your guide to a better, stronger mind:
- An Excursion of Change:

"Mind Over Issue: The Force of Yoga" isn't simply an aid; it's a challenge to carry on with an existence of mental clearness, close to home flexibility, and a solid, spry cerebrum.

It's an update that the ability to change your psychological and close to home state is inside your span.

Something other than an aide, "Mind Over Issue" is your guide to dominating the exceptional impact of yoga on your cerebrum.

It's your encouragement to take advantage of the significant wellspring of mental lucidity, profound prosperity, and versatile cerebrum wellbeing.

Your excursion to dominating the force of yoga starts here.

2. The Cerebrum Body Framework: Yoga's Significant Mental Advantages"

- The Cerebrum Body Framework: Yoga's Significant Mental Advantages"
- Association:

Yoga isn't just a progression of actual stances; it's an excursion into the perplexing association among the brain and body.

"The Cerebrum Body Platform" dives profound into this relationship, uncovering the manners by which yoga can fit and revive your psychological and close to home scene.

- An Excursion of Self-Investigation:

Yoga fills in as a significant device for self-investigation, driving you on a way of inward revelation.

This book is your confidant friend on this excursion, empowering you to investigate the limitless capability of your psyche, tap into its most profound breaks, and saddle the insight it holds.

- Close to home Flexibility and Stress Authority:

In a world full of stressors, yoga gives a safe-haven close to home strength.

"The Cerebrum Body Framework" acquaints you with yoga's surprising skill to oversee pressure, develop close to home prosperity, and sustain profound flexibility.

It's a pathway to profound harmony and inward quiet.

- Upgraded Mental Capability and Mental Clearness:

Yoga goes past quieting the psyche; it improves mental capability and mental clearness.

The book investigates how yoga tones your intellectual capacities, upgrades concentration and focus, and enhances inventive reasoning.

Your entrance to a psyche works at its pinnacle potential.

- Cerebrum Wellbeing and Brain adaptability:

Yoga isn't just about mental prosperity; it's about the strength of your mind.

"The Cerebrum Body Framework" reveals the manners by which yoga upholds brain adaptability, the mind's surprising ability to adjust and overhaul itself.

- It's your guide to a strong, coordinated mind:
- A Way to Change:

"The Cerebrum Body Platform: Yoga's Significant Mental Advantages" isn't simply an aid;

it's an encouragement to carry on with an existence set apart by mental clearness, profound flexibility, and a solid, deft mind.

It's an update that the ability to change your psychological and profound state is inside your grip.

Something beyond an aide, "The Mind Body Framework" is your guide to dominating the inconceivable effect of yoga on your psychological prosperity.

It's your challenge to take advantage of the significant wellspring of mental lucidity, profound versatility, and strong cerebrum wellbeing.

Your excursion to opening the significant mental advantages of yoga starts here.

Chapter 6:

Backing to Flourish
Yoga-Injected Sustenance
for Prosperity

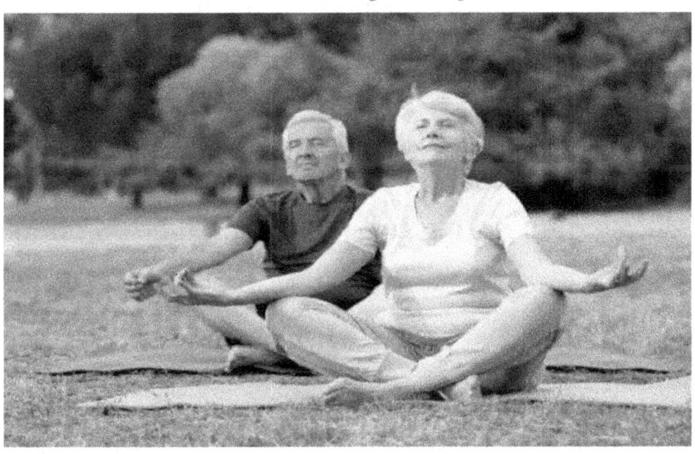

In a world loaded up with steady difficulties and turmoil, where prosperity frequently appears to be tricky, "Backing to Flourish:

Yoga-Implanted Sustenance for Prosperity" arises as a help.

This extensive aide reveals the significant collaboration among yoga and sustenance, offering a guide to get by as well as to flourish in each feature of life really.

- The Combination of Yoga and Sustenance:

Yoga and sustenance are not discrete substances; they are entwined components of all encompassing prosperity.

"Backing to Flourish" digs into this combination, uncovering the manners by which yoga can be incorporated into your way to deal with sustenance to help your physical, close to home, and mental success.

- An Excursion to Completeness:

Yoga is a training that goes past the mat; it stretches out to your plate and your way of life.

This book is your sidekick on an excursion toward completeness, welcoming you to investigate the comprehensive component of prosperity that emerges from the transaction of yoga and sustenance.

- Actual Prosperity and Essentialness:

Yoga-injected sustenance is your key to actual prosperity and endless imperativeness.

"Backing to Flourish" gives experiences into how the right sustenance decisions can upgrade your actual wellbeing, support your energy levels, and advance in general imperativeness.

- Close to home Strength and Happiness:

Sustenance isn't just about actual food; it assumes a crucial part in close to home strength.

This book digs into the profound sustenance given by a fair eating regimen and careful eating, cultivating close to home balance and a feeling of happiness.

- Mental Clearness and Innovativeness:

Yoga-mixed sustenance hones intellectual capacities and upgrades innovativeness.

The book investigates the manners by which feeding your body with the right food varieties can help mental clearness, fixation, and invigorate innovative reasoning. Your way to a psyche is clear and imaginative.

- A Recipe for Change:

"Backing to Flourish: Yoga-Implanted Sustenance for Prosperity" isn't simply an aide; it's a challenge to carry on with an existence set apart by prosperity, essentialness, and a significant feeling of completeness.

It's an update that the ability to change your life, beginning with your sustenance decisions, is inside your grip.

Something beyond an aide, "Backing to Flourish" is your guide to dominating the combination of yoga and sustenance.

It's your challenge to take advantage of the significant cooperative energy that exists between the two, preparing for an existence of imperativeness, close to home strength, and mental clearness.

Your excursion to flourishing through yoga-implanted sustenance starts here.

2. Food as Medication: Supplement Rich, Yoga-Roused Recipes"

In our current reality where the high speed of life frequently detaches us from the fundamental wellspring of prosperity — our food, "Food as Medication:

Supplement Rich, Yoga-Propelled Recipes" arises as a manual for eating as well as sustaining your body, psyche, and soul.

This extensive cookbook divulges a comprehensive way to deal with nourishment, wedding the insight of yoga with supplement rich recipes that act as both food and medication.

- Yoga's Effect on Sustenance:

Yoga and nourishment are characteristically connected, framing a strong mix for prosperity. "Food as Medication" dives into this association, uncovering how yoga can rouse your dietary decisions, prompting a better, more healthy lifestyle.

- An Excursion into Healthy Eating:

This cookbook isn't just about recipes; it's an excursion into healthy eating roused by yoga's standards of equilibrium and care.

"Food as Medication" welcomes you to investigate the significant association between your plate and your prosperity.

- Actual Wellbeing and Essentialness:

Supplement rich, yoga-roused recipes act as your key to actual wellbeing and limitless imperativeness.

This book gives experiences into how the right food varieties can upgrade your actual prosperity, help your energy levels, and advance by and large essentialness.

- Close to home Strength and Internal Harmony:

Sustaining your body with the right food sources goes past the physical; it adds to profound flexibility and inward harmony.

"Food as Medication" investigates the profound sustenance given by a decent eating regimen and careful eating, cultivating close to home harmony and a feeling of satisfaction.

- Mental Lucidity and Inventiveness:

Yoga-roused recipes feed your body as well as upgrade mental clearness and animate inventiveness.

This book reveals the manners by which appropriate sustenance can hone intellectual capacities, help fixation, and invigorate imaginative reasoning.

- Your way to a psyche is clear and imaginative:
- A Recipe for All encompassing Prosperity:

"Food as Medication: Supplement Rich, Yoga-Motivated Recipes" isn't simply a cookbook;

it's a challenge to have an existence set apart by prosperity, essentialness, and a significant feeling of completeness.

It's an update that the ability to change your life, beginning with your dietary decisions, is inside your grip.

- Something other than a cookbook, "Food as Medication" is your guide to dominating the combination of yoga and sustenance.

It's your challenge to take advantage of the significant cooperative energy that exists between the two, preparing for an existence of essentialness, profound versatility, and mental clearness.

Your excursion to sustaining your body and soul through yoga-roused recipes starts here.

Chapter 7:

Yoga, All things considered Embracing Day to day Practice

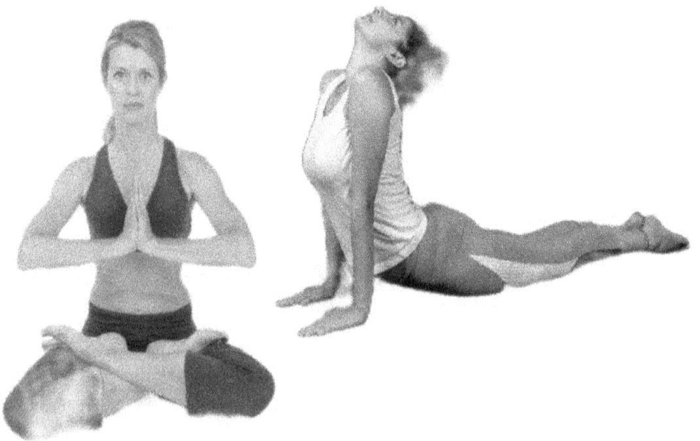

Yoga, All effects considered Embracing Day to day Practice" In the hurricane of our day to day routines, where scores, stress, and steady movement appear to overwhelm,"

- Yoga, All effects considered Embracing Day to day Practice" arises as a primer for constantly coordinate the extraordinary force of yoga into your ordinary presence:

This book uncovers the significant effect of yoga when it's not confined to the mat yet lived at the times between breaths.

Yoga history Mat Yoga is not just about breaking dramatically on a mat; it's a life. " Yoga, In actuality"

digs into the craft of integrating yoga norms into your day to day schedules, aiding you with encountering its enchantment in each aspect of your life.

- An All encompassing Way to deal with Health This book is not just about stations; it's tied in with embracing a comprehensive way to deal with substance:

" Yoga, In actuality" welcomes you to probe the different rudiments of yoga, including care, breathwork, and reflection, and what they can emphatically mean for your cerebral and close to home equilibrium.

Factual Imperativeness and Substance Everyday yoga practice adds to factual imperativeness and in general substance.

The book gives bits of knowledge into how integrating yoga stretches, works out, and careful developments into your everyday schedule can prompt expanded factual good and a dynamic, vigorous life.

Profound Versatility and Internal Congruity Yoga is not just about factual stations; it's an integral asset to support profound strength and internal concordance.

" Yoga, In actuality" investigates how yoga's cerebral and close to home angles can help you with overseeing pressure, encourage profound balance, and develop internal harmony.

- Mental Lucidity and Concentration The act of yoga is not confined to the body; it improves internal simplicity and hones your attention:

The book uncovers how yoga norms and care strategies can lift internal capability, further develop focus, and amp imaginative logic.

An Actuality of Equilibrium and Satisfaction " Yoga, All effects considered Embracing Everyday Practice" is not simply an assistant;

it's a stimulant to have an actuality set piecemeal by equilibrium, imperativeness, and satisfaction. It's an update that the capability to change your life, both authentically and intellectually, is inside your range. commodity beyond an assistant,"

- Yoga, All effects considered" is your companion to making yoga a necessary piece of your day to day presence:

It's your stimulant to encounter the significant effect of yoga in each alternate, cultivating a day to day actuality set piecemeal by imperativeness, profound versatility, and internal simplicity. Your excursion to embracing day to day yoga practice, in actuality, starts then.

2. Practice It Day to day: Incorporating Yoga into Your Ordinary Daily schedule"

In the midst of the rushing about of current life, where time is a valuable product and requests won't ever stop, "Practice It Day to day:

- Coordinating Yoga into Your Ordinary Daily schedule" remains as a directing light:

This exhaustive aide uncovers the extraordinary force of yoga when it turns into a fundamental piece of your day to day existence.

- Yoga as a Lifestyle:

Yoga isn't simply an action restricted to a particular overall setting; it's a lifestyle.

"Practice It Day to day" dives into the specialty of consistently meshing yoga into your everyday schedules, changing the unremarkable into the remarkable.

- All encompassing Health in Day to day Living:

This book isn't exclusively about asanas; it's tied in with embracing an all encompassing way to deal with prosperity in your regular routine.

"Practice It Everyday" welcomes you to investigate the different aspects of yoga, including care, breathwork, and reflection, and how they can emphatically impact your psychological and close to home equilibrium.

- Actual Strength and Energy:

Everyday yoga practice adds to actual strength and by and large dynamic quality.

The book offers experiences into how consolidating yoga stretches, works out, and careful developments into your everyday schedule can prompt better actual wellbeing and a daily existence loaded up with energy.

- Profound Flexibility and Internal Tranquility:

Yoga isn't just about actual stances; it's an incredible asset for supporting close to home flexibility and internal quietness.

"Practice It Everyday" investigates how yoga's psychological and close to home aspects can assist you with overseeing pressure, develop profound balance, and sustain inward harmony.

- Mental Lucidity and Concentration:

The act of yoga rises above the physical; it improves mental lucidity and hones your concentration.

The book uncovers how yoga standards and care methods can lift mental capability, further develop fixation, and invigorate inventive reasoning.

- An Existence of Concordance and Satisfaction:

"Practice It Day to day: Incorporating Yoga into Your Regular Daily Schedule" isn't simply an aid; it's a challenge to carry on with an existence set apart by congruity, essentialness, and satisfaction.

It's an update that the ability to change your life, both truly and intellectually, is inside your grip.

Something other than an aide, "Practice It Everyday" is your guide to making yoga an intrinsic piece of your day to day presence.

It's your encouragement to encounter the significant effect of yoga in each second, cultivating a day to day existence set apart by imperativeness, close to home flexibility, and mental clearness.

Your excursion to coordinating everyday yoga practice into your life starts here.

Chapter 8:

Practice It Day to day Incorporating Yoga into Your Ordinary Daily schedule

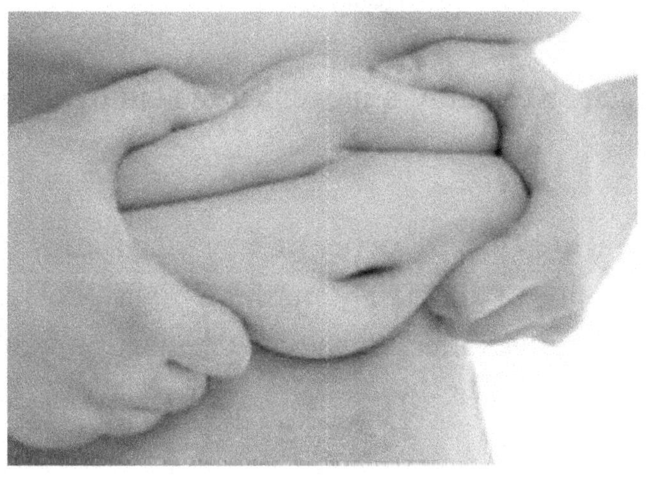

In the midst of the hurrying around of current life, where time is a valuable product and

Requests won't ever stop, "Practice It Day to day: Coordinating Yoga into Your Regular Daily schedule" remains as a directing light.

This thorough aide uncovers the extraordinary force of yoga when it turns into a necessary piece of your day to day existence.

- Yoga as a Lifestyle:

Yoga isn't simply a movement bound to a particular general setting;

it's a lifestyle. "Practice It Everyday" digs into the specialty of flawlessly meshing yoga into your day to day schedules, changing the unremarkable into the remarkable.

- All encompassing Health in Day to day Living:

This book isn't exclusively about asanas; it's tied in with embracing an all encompassing way to deal with prosperity in your regular routine.

"Practice It Everyday" welcomes you to investigate the different aspects of yoga, including care, breathwork, and reflection, and how they can decidedly impact your psychological and close to home equilibrium.

- Actual Strength and Dynamic quality:

Everyday yoga practice adds to actual strength and by and large dynamic quality.

The book offers experiences into how integrating yoga stretches, works out, and careful developments into your everyday schedule can prompt better actual wellbeing and a day to day existence loaded up with energy.

- Profound Strength and Inward Serenity:

Yoga isn't just about actual stances; it's an amazing asset for supporting profound versatility and inward peacefulness.

"Practice It Everyday" investigates how yoga's psychological and close to home aspects can assist you with overseeing pressure, develop profound harmony, and support inward harmony.

- Mental Lucidity and Concentration:

The act of yoga rises above the physical; it improves mental lucidity and hones your concentration.

The book uncovers how yoga standards and care strategies can lift mental capability, further develop fixation, and animate innovative reasoning.

- An Existence of Congruity and Satisfaction:

"Practice It Day to day: Coordinating Yoga into Your Regular Daily schedule" isn't simply an aide;

it's a challenge to have an existence set apart by concordance, essentialness, and satisfaction.

It's an update that the ability to change your life, both truly and intellectually, is inside your grip.

Something beyond an aide, "Practice It Day to day" is your guide to making yoga an intrinsic piece of your everyday presence.

It's your challenge to encounter the significant effect of yoga in each second, encouraging a day to day existence set apart by essentialness, profound strength, and mental lucidity.

Your excursion to coordinating day to day yoga practice into your life starts here.

1. Living the Yogi Way: Yoga's Basic beliefs forever"

In a world that frequently tests our qualities and standards, "Living the Yogi Way: Yoga's Basic Beliefs Forever" arises as a guiding light.

This far reaching guide uncovers the immortal insight of yoga, giving an outline to incorporating its fundamental beliefs into each part of your life.

- Yoga as a Lifestyle:
- Yoga is something other than actual stances; it's a lifestyle:

"Living the Yogi Way" digs into the core of yoga reasoning, stressing that its guiding principle stretches out a long ways past the mat, impacting your everyday decisions, communications, and generally prosperity.

- The Core values:

This book uncovers the essential standards of yoga, including sympathy, honesty, peacefulness, and self-restraint, among others.

"Living the Yogi Way" welcomes you to investigate how these standards can be your ethical compass, directing your activities and choices.

- Close to home Flexibility and Sympathy:

Yoga's fundamental beliefs go past oneself; they support profound flexibility and compassion.

"Living the Yogi Way" investigates how embracing these qualities can assist you with overseeing pressure, develop profound balance, and extend how you might interpret others' points of view.

- Mental Clearness and Internal Concordance:

The act of yoga isn't restricted to the body; it improves mental clearness and encourages internal agreement.

The book uncovers how yoga standards and care strategies can hone your concentration, work on your focus, and clear the way to internal harmony.

- An Existence of Uprightness and Satisfaction:

"Living the Yogi Way: Yoga's Basic beliefs forever" isn't simply an aide; it's a challenge to have an existence set apart by trustworthiness, compassion, and satisfaction.

It's an update that the insight of yoga's guiding principle gives serious areas of strength for exploring the intricacies of life.

Something other than an aide, "Living the Yogi Way" is your guide to making yoga's fundamental beliefs a necessary piece of your everyday presence.

It's your challenge to encounter the significant effect of living in arrangement with these standards, encouraging a daily existence set apart by trustworthiness, profound flexibility, and mental lucidity.

Your excursion to living the Yogi way starts here.

Conclusion :

- **Conclude Embracing the Concordance Inside"**

As we venture through the powerful embroidery of life, continually looking for equilibrium, meaning, and a more profound comprehension of our reality, we wind up at the finish of this extraordinary investigation.

"Embracing the Concordance Inside" fills in as a summit, a reflection on the significant excursion we have attempted to adjust our internal and external universes.

- The Embodiment of Yoga:

All through this book, we have dove into the embodiment of yoga, rising above the actual practice to embrace its comprehensive way of thinking.

Yoga isn't bound to stances on a mat; a lifestyle entices us to adjust our qualities, activities, and internal world with the congruity of the universe.

- Embracing Solidarity and Equilibrium:

In these pages, we have disclosed the insight of yoga's fundamental beliefs, lessons that rise above social and strict limits.

We have come to figure out that embracing sympathy, honesty, and peacefulness cultivates close to home flexibility, compassion, and a feeling of solidarity with every single residing being.

- Mental Lucidity and Inward Harmony:

Yoga isn't just about the adaptability of the body; it's about the adaptability of the brain.

Our investigation has demonstrated the way that psychological clearness, concentration, and innovativeness can be supported through care and the act of yoga standards. This psychological clearness clears the way to internal harmony.

- A Daily existence Lined up with Values:

"Embracing the Concordance Inside" has been a challenge to have an existence lined up with values.

Yoga reasoning fills in as our directing compass, assisting us with pursuing decisions that reverberate with our most profound standards, prompting an existence of honesty, sympathy, and satisfaction.

- Your Continuous Excursion:

As we finish up this excursion, it's memorable's essential that embracing the concordance inside isn't an objective however a ceaseless interaction.

We are in various ways, very interesting and continually advancing.

The insight of yoga fills in as an immortal aide, supporting us as we explore life's difficulties and delights.

- Determination: A Fresh start:

This determination denotes a fresh start, a continuous excursion of self-disclosure, development, and change.

It is an encouragement to convey the insight of yoga with you, permitting it to inject each part of your reality, cultivating solidarity, balance, mental clearness, and uprightness.

Something other than a book, "Embracing the Concordance Inside" is an update that the ability to adjust your internal and external universes is inside your grip.

It's a guide to carrying on with a day to day existence set apart by solidarity, balance, close to home flexibility, and mental lucidity.

Your excursion to embracing the concordance inside proceeds, a significant investigation that improves your life's embroidery.